Antioxidants

A Simple Method to Increase Brain Power, Strengthen Your Immune System and Reverse the Aging Process

Ruth Logan

CONTENTS

1   Introduction   6

2   Benefits to Antioxidants   9

3   Types of Antioxidants   12

4   Top 7 Antioxidants NOT to miss out on   24

5   Why Is It Important to Win the Free Radical Fight?   30

6   Simple Ways to Sneak Antioxidants into Your Diet   34

7   The Top 3 Ways to Drink Your Antioxidants   42

8   Treasure Hunt – Find Antioxidant Food Sources in a Fun   46
     and Easy Way

9   Top 10 Cheap, Hassle Free and Antioxidant Rich Meals   53

10   Food & Drink-Free Antioxidant Boosters   58

11   Super Antioxidant Breakfast, Lunch and Dinner Options   61

12   Conclusion   63

     About the Author   65

     More Books by Ruth Logan   66

ANTIOXIDANTS

ANTIOXIDANTS

INTRODUCTION

At every corner that we turn, there always seems to be something new and unique trying to lure us into trying new 'fads'. This is especially true for things that are trying to attack our health. Whether it is consuming excessive amounts of sugar, having high cholesterol or a myriad of diseases we can't seem to count, everything is out to get us. Unfortunately, there is a widely unknown villain out there trying to damage our living cells. These pesky villains are selfish molecules known as "free radicals". Of course, with every villain there is a hero to stop them dead in their tracks. That hero is the focus of this book; Antioxidants. Before we can truly understand antioxidants and learn how to sneak them into our diets, we must first understand why we need them.

As I mentioned above, the reasons why we need antioxidants is to counter the impact of what free radicals do to our cells. So, what exactly do free radicals do to our cells? The science behind the answer can be a bit tricky to understand, so let's try to explain it as simple as possible. Free Radicals are molecules that want what other molecules have; stability. For a molecule to become stable, all of its electrons in its outer shell must be paired off. To illustrate, think about a group of high schoolers all going to prom. I suspect you are imagining that most of them are paired off and feel "happy". But then you notice one of the teens. There is one kid named Freddy but everyone calls him Freddy the Free Radical. Freddy does not want to be alone so he goes seeking a partner. He is so desperate, that he even tries to take someone else's partner! How inconsiderate of our friend Freddy. Free Radicals try a similar move with our happy healthy cells.

Free Radicals are molecules that have unpaired electrons. They are looking to take electrons or make bonds with other molecules even if that means being inconsiderate like our friend Freddy and trying to rip happy molecules apart. However, these bad guys were not always such trouble makers. They were once stable molecules themselves. So, what happened? Oxidation happened!

What is Oxidation? To put it simply, oxidation is the loss or increase of electrons in a molecule. When this process occurs in our cells and tissues, it's called "oxidative stress". So, what exactly is it that causes oxidation? Unfortunately there is not one exact culprit. There are a lot of various different factors that cause oxidation such as the following:

- Stress

- Poor Diet

- Radiation

- Drugs

- Pollution

- Infection

- Aging

- Injury

Now keep in mind that this is not a complete list. There are many other oxidation factors as well. So now we know what causes oxidation and we also know that free radicals are a product of oxidation, but now we need to figure out two things. What is it that makes free radicals so dangerous and what effects do these free radicals have on our bodies?

Think back to the illustration mentioned before. Remember Freddy?

Let's say he was successful in taking away a person who had already bonded with someone else. What would happen? Besides some hurt feelings nothing would really change, there still would be only one person looking for a bond and one newly formed bond. This is a potential outcome with molecules as well, though not the only outcome. One end result of a free radical stealing an electron away from an already made molecular bond is that the free radical just ends up stealing an electron and not making any bonds with a molecule. This then transforms two, once happy molecules, into two miserable free radicals. Just think! What if this process continued like this? Each time a free radical steals an electron away to become stable, two unstable molecules take its place! This chain reaction is very dangerous and could cause serious damage to any tissue and also cause a myriad of other issues that include:

- Cancer

- Arthritis

- Swelling

- Autoimmune Disease

- Heart Disease

- Neurological Disease

- Pulmonary Disease

- Nephropathy

- And over 80 more!

Free radicals sound terrifying! They are always popping up in are cells, willing to attack any part of our bodies, and can cause some serious illness and even disease. Should we panic and give up now? No! Why? We have antioxidants! They are in almost every healthy food and can stop free radicals from wreaking havoc in our bodies. Our next step is figuring out how antioxidants work and what are their benefits.

BENEFITS TO ANTIOXIDANTS

Antioxidants are powerful molecules that can help neutralize the effects of free radicals, but how? Free radicals just want to be like everyone else and become stable, they make bonds to achieve this. Antioxidants are molecules that have an abundance of extra electrons that free radicals can use to become balanced. The best part about this is that no antioxidants are harmed in this process. The unstable molecules become stable, causing no other disturbances and the antioxidants do not become unstable molecules. Everyone wins but more importantly, you win! Let's go over the 3 ways antioxidants help against free radicals and keeping your cells healthy.

1. **Neutralizing**: Imagine you had a friend with a nail stuck in their hand. The pain is excruciating and every second you waste, the risk of infection grows greater and greater. What would you do first to help them? Would you sit them down, go on the internet and look up ways to stop the pain? Maybe you would try to put some healing cream on the hand and over the nail to stop the bleeding. Would this work? Of course not! Any sane person is going to get to the root of the problem first and take the nail out of the hand first, or take them to the hospital for the same result. Antioxidants work in a similar fashion. Before trying to heal any of the damaged cells, antioxidants first stabilize any of the free radicals, so that they don't cause any more damage.

2. **Healing**: After antioxidants stabilizes the free radicals, they move on to healing the damaged cells left by the free radicals. Replacing stolen electrons back to the molecules and stopping the chain of oxidation.

3.   **Preventing**: Antioxidants also prevent future free radicals from rearing their ugly heads again. They also prevent many of the problems we've discuss before, such as heart problems, skin problems, and many others but we will discuss these more in depth later.

There are many benefits from antioxidants, one of them includes preventing heart disease which is so deadly that it results in an average of 1 death every 36 seconds. The American Heart Association says, "Oxidation of low-density bad cholesterol is important in the development of fatty buildups in the arteries. This process, called atherosclerosis, can lead to heart attacks and strokes. Increasing evidence suggests that these bad cholesterol oxidations and its biological effects can be prevented by increasing antioxidants — both in the diet and in supplements." In 1993, Harvard University researchers reported that supplemental doses of vitamin E actually reduced the risk of heart disease by as much as 54 percent! We will talk more about the various different kinds of antioxidants in the next chapter.

Can antioxidants reduce the likelihood of cancer in humans? This is an important question for us to know the answer to since most people either have cancer or know of someone who has cancer. Statistics show that one in every three people will get cancer, one of those four will die from it. Antioxidants have been proven to help breast cancer. Experts have said that if every woman in America started upping there consumption of antioxidants, then within a few years the breast cancer rate in this country would drastically decline. One study has shown that 200 micrograms of a specific antioxidant would cut the rate of lung cancer by 34% and prostate cancer by 69%. The short answer is 'Yes'.

Antioxidants are very important for all of us. They help us guard against disease, by strengthening and protecting our immune systems. Did you know that antioxidants may even help us live longer! Free radicals cause aging, and antioxidants in high enough quantities can heal that damaged cells and in turn, slow the aging process. How much life can some antioxidants give us? Just a few milligrams of those beneficial vitamins a day can give us on average of 4 years of extra life!

A wonderful thing about antioxidants is that they are made naturally by our bodies. However, with the growing number of things that cause oxidation, our bodies don't produce enough natural antioxidants to keep going. We need to consume them to increase levels. The good news is some of the highest concentrations of various antioxidants are found in some of the most brightly colored fruits and vegetables, and most of us are fortunate to have easy access to these foods at our local grocery store. These include; carrots, red bell peppers, tomatoes, raspberries, numerous kinds of nuts, pomegranates, spinach and many more!

Now, we understand the importance of antioxidants, and the benefits they provide. Let's delve into all the different kinds of antioxidants, what foods they're in and how they specifically benefit our bodies.

TYPES OF ANTIOXIDANTS

There are lots of different kinds of antioxidants. Some of which we might already be familiar with, such as vitamin E, vitamin C, magnesium and zinc. There's a strong possibility that you haven't heard of some of the antioxidants I refer to in this book, please don't be deterred, this is completely normal. I plan on covering the other types of antioxidants, what they do, the recommended intake, what foods you can find them in and creative ways you can sneak them into your diet.

Let's start by looking at the most common types of antioxidants.

Vitamin A

What is it?

Vitamin A is found in three main forms: vitamin A1, vitamin A2 and vitamin A3.

What does it do?

Vitamin A is a powerful antioxidant that acts as a hormone in the body, affecting the expression of genes and thereby influencing phenotype. Retinol is the predominant active form of vitamin A found in the blood.

What is the recommended intake?

The intake of vitamin A varies according to the age and sex of whoever consumes it. Since vitamin A is available in several forms, the vitamin A content in foods is often measured as "retinol activity equivalents", or

RAEs for short. The intake for different ages are as followed:

- 0-6 months: 400mcg/day
- 7-12 months: 500mcg/day
- 1-3 years: 300 mcg/day
- 4-8 years: 400 mcg/day
- 9-13 years: 600 mcg/day
- 14+ years (male): 900 mcg/day
- 14+ years (female): 700 mcg/day
- 14-18 years (pregnancy): 750 mcg/day
- 14-18 years (lactation): 1,200 mcg/day
- 19-50 years (pregnancy): 770 mcg/day
- 19-50 years (lactation): 1,300 mcg/day.

There are consequences for not taking in enough vitamin A, these include night blindness, higher susceptibility to infections and follicular hyperkeratosis. There are lots of benefits to vitamin A, one big one is lowering cancer risk. Higher intakes of vitamin A from fruits and vegetables are associated with a lower risk of lung cancer. Other vitamin supplements have not shown the same results.

Among younger men, diets rich in vitamin A may play a protective role against prostate cancer, according to a study conducted by the Harvard School of Public Health's Department of Nutrition. Vitamin A has also been shown to have an inverse association with the development of colon cancer in the Japanese population.

How can it help?

Vitamin A helps in treating type 2 diabetes, preventing asthma, as well giving us healthy living skin and hair. Retinoic acid, a derivative of vitamin A, has been found to normalize blood sugar in diabetic mice. In preventing asthma, the risks of developing asthma are lower in people who consume a high amount of vitamin A. And don't all of us want healthy looking skin and hair! Vitamin A plays an important role in the growth of all bodily tissues, including skin and hair, and is also needed for the production of sebum, the oil that helps maintain levels of moisture in the skin and hair.

Where can I find it?

Okay we get it, vitamin A is good for us but how do we get this precious antioxidant into our bodies! Ready-made retinol, the active form of vitamin A, can only be obtained from animal sources. The richest sources of retinol are:

- Herring in oils with chives and onion

- Liver

- Fatty fish (like herring and salmon)

- Fish oils

- Butter

- Milk

- Cheese

- Eggs.

Plant-based foods contain the precursor antioxidant form of vitamin A, carotenoids, which are then converted to retinol in the body. This antioxidant is also an orange pigment and contributes to the color of certain fruits and vegetables. Rich sources of vitamin A include orange plant foods such as butternut squash, papaya, apricots, cantaloupe, pumpkin and carrots. Other plant foods, such as broccoli, dark leafy green vegetables, zucchini and peppers are also a rich source of vitamin A, with an array of pigments combining to create the bright colors seen in vegetables and fruits.

Getting this antioxidant in our bodies should not be too hard. Who wouldn't want a fresh omelet in the morning with eggs and cheese? Or maybe some nicely roasted broccoli or squash? Of course, there will be some foods we are not so thrilled about eating but we can't let that stop us! With a little bit of creativeness and some seasoning, any food can be transformed into something delicious and healthy!

Lutein

What is it?

Lutein is called a carotenoid vitamin and is related to vitamin A. Carotenoids are the pigments that give fruits and vegetables there bright colors.

What does it do?

Lutein is often known as the "eye vitamin". Many people use it to prevent eye diseases such as; age-related macular degeneration or AMD for short. Some studies have even shown that eating higher amounts of lutein can decrease the risk of developing cataracts.

What is the recommending intake?

For reducing the risk of cataracts and age-related macular degeneration (AMD): one should consume around 6 mg of lutein per day. People consuming 6.9 to 11.7 mg of lutein per day had the lowest risk of developing AMD and cataracts.

Where can I find it?

How can we get lutein in our body? Foods that tend to be rich in lutein include:

- Squash
- Zucchini
- Orange juice
- Kiwi fruit
- Grapes
- Orange pepper
- Corn
- Kale
- Spinach
- Broccoli

One way some people found to get lutein into their system is by making a delicious smoothie with, kale, grapes, kiwi, and orange juice. Zucchini over a nice steak is not only yummy but also good for you!

Lycopene

What is it?

Lycopene is a naturally occurring chemical that gives fruits and vegetables their beautiful red color. It, like lutein, is also a carotenoid.

What does it do?

People take lycopene for preventing heart disease, "hardening of the arteries" (atherosclerosis), and cancer of the prostate, breast, lung, bladder, ovaries, colon, and pancreas. Lycopene is also used for treating human papilloma virus (HPV) infection, which is a major cause of uterine cancer. Some people also use lycopene for cataracts and asthma. Are you noticing a trend? A lot of these antioxidant's benefits tend to overlap.

What is the recommended intake?

The appropriate dose of lycopene depends on several factors such as the user's age, health and several other conditions. At this time there is not enough scientific information to determine an appropriate range of doses for lycopene, bummer I know. Keep in mind that natural products are not always necessarily safe and dosages can be important. Be sure to follow relevant directions on product labels and consult your pharmacist or physician or other healthcare professional before using.

Where can we find it?

(Cooked) Tomatoes. That's the answer! Tomatoes are known to have high amounts of lycopene in them. Some other foods that have lycopene in them are:

- Pink grapefruits

- Watermelons

- Apricots

- Pink guavas

- Ketchup

Anytime we use tomato juice or put ketchup on a nice burger, we are consume high amounts of lycopene. This one isn't so tricky to get into our diets.

Vitamin C

What is it?

Vitamin C is the Golden Boy of antioxidants. It is known to help in a broad spectrum of problems and even allow us to live longer.

What does it do?

A better question may be, what does it not do? It has been shown to help in colds, true it may not literally cure it but taking vitamin C can reduce the risk of developing further complications, such as pneumonia and lung infections. Vitamin C is unique in that it's one of the nutrients that is sensitive to stress. It is normally one of the first antioxidants to leave the body in smokers, obese individuals, and alcoholics. Basically if you have vitamin C in you, odds are your overall health is going pretty good.

What is the recommended intake?

Most studies figured the use of 500 daily milligrams of vitamin C to achieve health results. That's much higher than the RDA of 70-90 milligrams a day for adults. To put that in prospective you would need to eat 63 apples to get the recommended intake for vitamin C. I don't know about you but I don't know of many people that throw down 63 apples a day.

So in this case, in order to get vitamin C inside you, a dietary supplement may be need to gain all the benefits. Some experts suggests taking 500 milligrams a day, in addition to eating five servings of fruits and vegetables. It is just not practical for anyone to eat as much food that is needed to gain 500 milligrams a day of vitamin C. Fortunately taking supplements for vitamin C has little to no risk since 2000 milligrams is still considered safe.

Where can we find it?

Vitamin C is can be found in a vast range of foods. Most people associate Vitamin C with citrus fruit, and they're right to do so. However, there are higher concentrations of Vitamin C in the following foods:

- Papaya
- Bell Peppers
- Broccoli
- Brussel Sprouts
- Strawberries
- Pineapple
- Oranges
- Kiwi Fruit

Selenium

What is it?

Selenium is an essential trace mineral important for cognitive function, a healthy immune system and if you are having troubles making a baby, selenium is the antioxidant for you! Selenium is shown to boost fertility in both men and women.

What does it do?

Selenium is involved in the production of prostaglandins in the body, which regulate inflammation and may reduce inflammation related to arthritis. A study out of the Netherlands has linked selenium intake to a lower risk of prostate cancer. Researchers tested the levels of selenium in the toenails of study participants, a marker that measures long-term selenium intake. The researchers found that the greater the level of selenium in the toenail, the lower the risk for prostate cancer in study participants. Who knew toenails could ever be so useful! Selenium also works in close conjunction with vitamin E as an antioxidant to prevent the formation of free radicals and in turn, may reduce the risk of skin cancer and prevent sunburn.

What is the recommended intake?

The Recommended Daily Allowance for selenium is 55 micrograms per day for adults. Pregnant and lactating women have a slightly higher need for selenium at 60 and 70 micrograms per day.

Selenium deficiency is something very rare worldwide, it often takes years to develop and is usually only found in regions with severely low selenium content in the soil. Several regions in China with low soil selenium content have eradicated deficiencies in the population through supplementation programs. Should you take Selenium supplements? That of course is up to you but living in America, unless you lived in a literal dump, you would have to try to not get your daily selenium intake since it is in so many different foods.

Where can we find it?

Selenium is in a lot of various Seafood but is also in some other foods at well. These include:

- Brazil nuts

- Halibut

- Tuna

- Oysters

- White rice (long grain)

- Lobster

- Sunflower seeds

- Eggs

- Whole wheat

We've already mentioned how we can use eggs in a multitude of different ways to incorporate them in our diets. One great way to crave hunger urges is to snack on sunflower seeds, they are cheap, healthy and tasty! Tuna is also on the list above along with whole wheat, so how about a nice tune sandwich for lunch? It is just as affordable as sunflower seeds but also just as yummy!

Vitamin E

Vitamin E is last on our list of common antioxidants but it is just as important as the rest.

What is it?

Vitamin E is an antioxidant which helps protect your cells from damage. This essential nutrient occurs naturally in many foods, is available as a dietary supplement, and sometimes is added to processed foods. Vitamin E is fat-soluble, which means your body stores and uses it as needed. Collectively, the term Vitamin E describes eight different compounds, but alpha-tocopherol is the most active in humans.

What does it do?

The lack of vitamin E has been directly linked to movement disorder (ataxia). Vitamin E also slows down worsening memory loss in people with moderately severe Alzheimer's disease. Keep in mind though that vitamin E has not been proven to prevent moving from mild memory problems to Alzheimer's disease. Vitamin E is very useful in dealing with cancer but in different way than other antioxidants. True, vitamin E seems to aid in reducing mortality in patients with bladder cancer but it also eases chemotherapy. Taking vitamin E or more specifically, alpha-tocopherol, before and after treatment with chemotherapy might reduce the risk of nerve damage.

Vitamin E is a great antioxidant for women as it has been shown that taking vitamin E for 2 days before and for 3 days after bleeding begins, it decreases pain severity, duration and reduce menstrual blood loss. This antioxidant is fantastic for all sorts of people including our older generation. Research suggest that increasing vitamin E intake in our diet is linked with improved physical performance and muscle strength.

There are numerous other benefits from vitamin E that include:

- Blood disorder

- Dementia

- Liver disease

- Parkinson's disease

- Kidney problems found in children

- Healing from laser eye surgery

- Combating sunburn

What is the recommended intake?

Dosing for vitamin E can be confusing since it hugely depends on what you are taking it for. Typically, the average dose in adults is 75 IU a day.

Where can we find it?

Vitamin E is found in many foods including vegetable oils, cereals, meat, poultry, eggs, fruits, vegetables, and wheat germ oil. It is also available as a supplement. Since this antioxidant is so abundant in so many foods, fitting it in your diet should be a piece a cake. Not a literal piece of cake though, more like a piece of broccoli!

That concludes my list of the most common types of antioxidants and true, they are all very good for you, but there are 7 super antioxidants that you don't not want to miss out on in the next chapter. Some of these are harder to find, but they are extremely powerful and beneficial. We've mentioned a couple in the book so far, but there are some that you might not be aware of.

TOP 7 ANTIOXIDANTS NOT TO MISS OUT ON

There is a seemingly endless list of antioxidants that all have different benefits and purposes. Still hidden away from the common public are 7 antioxidants that either do a multitude of things well or are extremely beneficial for specific things. One of these antioxidants we already mentioned previously but it's so good for you we have to mention it again is Flavonols.

Flavonols

The most abundant and commonly known flavonoid in this group is called quercetin, which is found in yellow onions, broccoli, scallions, kale, berries, apples and teas. Flavonoids are a group of compounds found in plants that make up a certain group of antioxidants.

Alpha-lipoic Acid (ALA)

This antioxidant is as useful to the brain as it is difficult for our brains to say it. Aside from its amazing free radical scavenging abilities, this powerful antioxidant is also great at other things, these include:

- Heavy metal chelator

- Enhancing insulin sensitivity

- Modifying gene expressions to reduce inflammation

Alpha-lipoic Acid is the only antioxidant that can be easily transported into your brain, which offers numerous benefits for people with brain diseases such as, dementia and Alzheimer's disease. ALA can also regenerate other antioxidants, like vitamins C and E and glutathione. This means that if your body has used up these antioxidants, ALA can help regenerate them. Just think this is the glue that keeps all the other antioxidants running in our bodies.

Resveratrol

Unlike other antioxidants resveratrol cannot be manufactured inside your body and must be obtained from antioxidant rich foods or potent antioxidant supplements. Resveratrol are found in certain fruits like grapes, red wine, vegetables and cocoa. This antioxidant can cross the barrier between your blood and your brain, providing protection for your nervous system and brain. Just like every other antioxidant; resveratrol provides free radical protection but it can also help with:

- Normalizing your anti-inflammatory responses

- Preventing Alzheimer's disease

- Lowering your blood pressure

- Inhibiting the spread of cancer, especially prostate cancer

- Keeping your heart healthy

- Improving the elasticity of your blood vessels

This antioxidant was dubbed the "fountain of youth" because it is so effective at warding off aging related diseases.

Astaxanthin

This antioxidant is on list due to its brilliant nutritional advantages. Astaxanthin is a marine carotenoid produce by the microalgae

Haematococcus Pluvialis. Try saying that 5 time fast! Astaxanthin is produced when the Haematococcus Pluvialis water supply dries up, to give itself protection from ultraviolet radiation. Astaxanthin is one of the strongest carotenoids in term of free radical scavenging. It is 14 times more powerful than vitamin E, 54 times more powerful than beta-carotene and 65 times more powerful than vitamin C.

Like resveratrol, it can also cross the blood-brain barrier AND the blood-retinal barrier. This is something that beta-carotene and lycopene cannot do. Astaxanthin is also more effective than other carotenoids at "singlet oxygen quenching," a particular type of oxidation caused by sunlight and various organic materials. Astaxanthin is 550 times more powerful than vitamin E and 11 times more powerful than beta-carotene at neutralizing this specific kind of oxidation. Astaxanthin is amazing at all kind of things trying to list them all would very difficult but we will mention the important ones, such as:

- Supporting your immune function

- Improving your cardiovascular health by reducing C-Reactive Proteins (CRP) and triglycerides, and increasing beneficial

- Protecting your eyes from cataracts, macular degeneration, and blindness

- Protecting your brain from dementia and Alzheimer's

- Reducing your risk of different types of cancer

- Promoting recovery from spinal cord and other central nervous system injuries

- Reducing inflammation from all causes, including arthritis and asthma

- Improving your endurance, workout performance, and recovery

- Relieving indigestion and reflux

- Helping stabilize your blood sugar, thereby protecting your kidneys

- Increasing sperm strength and sperm count and improving fertility

- Helping prevent sunburn and protecting you from damaging radiation effects

- Reducing oxidative damage to your DNA

Astaxanthin also helps in reducing symptoms of diseases, such as pancreatitis, multiple sclerosis, carpal tunnel syndrome, rheumatoid arthritis, Lou Gehrig's disease, Parkinson's disease and neurodegenerative diseases.

This miracle antioxidant isn't found in any food unfortunately but you can find supplements of this online or by talking to your local doctor.

Vitamin C

We have talked about vitamin C before but it is so important and beneficial it is worth mentioning again. Since we already discussed vitamin C previously, we are just going to mention a few things we haven't thus far. We already know that vitamin C battles oxidation by acting as a major electron donor, it also maintains optimal electron flow in your cells, and protects proteins, lipids, and other vital molecular elements in your body. No wonder vitamin C is known as the "grandfather" of antioxidants, it is battling, maintaining, and protecting other cells in your body! Just as a loving grandfather would do.

CoQ10 (Ubiquinone)

CoQ10 gets around, it is used by every cell in your body and is converted by your body to its reduced form, called ubiquinol. CoQ10 has been the subject of thousands of studies and is found to benefit us in a numerous, it also:

-   Helps produce more energy for your cells

-   Provides support for your heart health, immune system, and nervous system

-   Helps reduce the signs of normal aging

-   Helps maintain blood pressure levels within the normal range

If you're under 25 years old, your body can convert CoQ10 to ubiquinol without any difficulty. However, when you get older, your body becomes more and more challenged to convert the oxidized CoQ10 to ubiquinol. Therefore, you may need to take an ubiquinol supplement.

Glutathione

Sometimes our own bodies can produce its own antioxidants and there is no better one than glutathione. It is known as the "master antioxidant" because it is inside our cells and has the unique ability of maximizing the performance of all the other antioxidants, including vitamin C, vitamin E, CoQ10, alpha-lipoic acid, and even the fruits and vegetables and fruits that you eat every day.

Glutathione's main function is to protect your cells from oxidative and peroxidative damage. It is also very important for detoxification, energy utilization and preventing the diseases we associate with aging. Glutathione also gets rid of toxins from your cells and is a shield from the damaging effects of radiation, chemicals and environmental pollutants.

Unfortunately, our body's ability to produce glutathione declines as we get older. However, there are nutrients that can promote glutathione production, such as:

- Sulfur-rich foods (garlic, onions, parsley, etc.)

- Native whey protein

- Raw milk and eggs

- Organ and red meats

- Organic turmeric

- Healthy exercise

It is very important to practice methods that promote glutathione production but it is just as important to actively minimize the factors that cause its depletion. Chronic low level stress in one of the primary means by which glutathione vanishes from our bodies. Finding a way to reduce stress can be hard but it I can be done. It can be as simple as going outside more often, laughing with a few of your good friends, or reading. It is one of the most genuine steps you can take towards a healthy happy life.

WHY IS IT IMPORTANT TO WIN THE FREE RADICAL FIGHT?

As we mentioned before at the outset of this book, there are many things that can harm our body, Free Radicals lead the way. Fortunately, we have learned about the tools we have to fight against these horrible menaces. We've learned about the "who, what, where, and why" of antioxidants.

The "who"? Easy! The star of show; antioxidants. We also learned that there are many different kinds of antioxidants such as:

-   Vitamin A

-   Vitamin C

-   Lutein

-   Vitamin E

-   Lycopene

-   Selenium

And some of the heavy hitters such as:

-   CoQ10

-   Vitamin C (again)

-   Astaxanthin

-   Alpha-lipoic Acid (ALA)

-   Resveratrol

-   Glutathione

We learned "what" these antioxidants do for our health. One of the biggest things we have found is how much antioxidants help with preventing cancer. They do this by giving their electrons away to free radicals and damaged cells so that they can become stable. They do this whilst not becoming free radicals themselves. Antioxidants also help with a multitude of other things. Mental health is one that kept coming up. Some antioxidants have shown to help restore and prevent some damage to our brains that has been caused by aging. Other antioxidants help with our eyesight and giving us healthier skin. The best antioxidants though are the ones that affect others in our body. Examples such as glutathione, are the parents of antioxidants as they keep all the other ones in our body going strong.

The "where" was an important thing we learned since, if we can't get these amazing antioxidants in our body then they would provide no use for us. Most of the foods that contain antioxidants tend to overlap. A lot of fruits and vegetables contain one or more kinds of antioxidants. Same is true for nuts, eggs, some meats, wheat and many other foods. Did you know that some of these foods with specific antioxidants, are healthier for you if eaten with other specific foods? One example of this are tomatoes and brussel sprouts. By themselves they are very good for you, but together they are 10 times more powerful. Another great way we haven't talked about to sneak some of these antioxidants into our body is through tea. Tea drinkers rejoice! Many kinds of tea have some form of food or chemicals that release antioxidants into our bodies. One tip to make sure you are getting the most out of your tea, is to dip your tea bag in and out of the cup so that all of the good stuff in the tea bag gets released into our cup. Make sure it's well brewed.

I know what you are thinking, what if I don't like or simply cannot have some of the foods mentioned? If you don't like some of the foods, an easy way to fix that is to mix things up. Don't like some vegetables? Maybe find a different way to cook and season them so that you are eating healthy but also enjoying it as well. Another tip when cooking food with antioxidants is to never boil the food. Boiling the food kills most of the antioxidants and makes eating it for health purposes pointless. What if you have allergies that stop you from eating some of the foods mentioned? No worries! Most of the antioxidants have supplements that you can attain. Just remember that in most cases, nothing is better than the antioxidants that the earth has provided for us.

We have all this information but how can we get motivated to use it in our day to day lives? "Why" is it important to win this battle against antioxidants? Forget the fact that our lives may be at risk, the main reason we should want to win this fight is be but more importantly to feel healthy!

Many people already suffer from health issues, if this includes you, then there is no time to wait. Your body can't do it on its own, not anymore. With all the pollution, unhealthy food, and a growing number of things that keeps our bodies down in the dumps, we have to help our bodies in the fight against free radicals. There is no such thing as starting to late, but the longer you wait the more free radicals are running rampant in our cells causing all kinds of damage.

If you're one of the fortunate ones that doesn't have any serious health concerns at the moment, that's great, but it's likely that at some stage your health will deteriorate, be it the flu or even a sickness bug. If you can, be proactive. The sooner you start putting antioxidants into your body the easier it will be to stick to it as you get older and it will also lower your risk of getting many diseases.

I understand that it is hard, we all live very busy lives and sometimes it's easier to go to a fast food chain and ignore the healthy route. Just remember that rarely anything worth having ever comes easily. Try to do what's 'right' as opposed to what's 'easy'. The more we incorporate antioxidants into our diet, the easier it will become for us to stay in the habit. Why stop there though? Share this book and its information with your friends and family. Inform other people about free radicals and antioxidants because sadly, most people have no idea. How can they fight against something they don't know there fighting? The more we learn to love living a healthier lifestyle, the more likely we'll be able to help other people fight the good fight against free radicals with our hero, antioxidants..

SIMPLE WAYS TO SNEAK ANTIOXIDANTS INTO YOUR DIET

It seems like every day we are bombarded with a new list of foods we should or should not eat. Some foods are too high in fat, while some are too low in fat. One day we should eat green foods, and the next we should eat only orange food. I have not even mentioned all the foods that were once deemed healthy, but now are apparently bad. How are we supposed to understand all this jargon? Don't you wish there was a simple solution?

Well, I am here to tell you that there is. The one rule when it comes to incorporating healthy food, rich in antioxidants into your diet is:

EAT REAL FOOD!

Is it that simple, you might ask? That can't be right? Hundreds of books are written every day on the subject; whole careers are made out of creating healthy diets.

But that is what I am saying – it is all a façade! All you have to do is eat REAL FOOD. You do not have to take 100 supplements; you do not have to buy expensive health food brands.

If you simply eat real food – food where you can pronounce the ingredients, and you know what the ingredients are – you will increase your antioxidant consumption the vast majority of time.

The important thing to remember here is this DOES NOT have to be COMPLICATED! You can eat fast food, but choose the options that are the least artificial. Go ahead, buy some packaged foods if you must – we do not have the inclination to cook dinner every night – just read the label so you understand what it is you are eating.

Do not worry; I am not going to leave you with just the vague (but true) instruction to EAT REAL FOOD. In food, antioxidants most often come in the form of vitamins, flavonoids, carotenoids, and minerals.

I will next show you five easy ways to sneak antioxidants into your diet. No rule book necessary

Fresh Vegetables

Fresh vegetables are loaded with vitamins, and unsurprisingly, antioxidants. There are so many ways to sneak fresh vegetables into your meals it's hard to know where to start.

The easiest way I find to increase my vegetable intake is to make them readily available. Cut up a variety of vegetables in easy to eat, finger sized, portions. Fill a snack container with carrot sticks, cut up sweet peppers, celery sticks, and broccoli and keep it at your desk or workspace while you work. Often when our minds are busy working, our hands will mindlessly snack at whatever is available. Too often, it is fatty chips or chemical-laden pre-packaged snacks that are the closest at hand. If you have a small container of easy to eat veggies within arm's reach, you are certain to consume more of these antioxidant rich foods.

If munching on raw vegetables doesn't sound like a good alternative to the nearest vending machine, buy or prepare a low fat dip to go with them. If you dip your veggies in a rich, creamy dip you will get the decadence of the snacks you are used to, but you will be adding to your antioxidants and fighting sickness at the same time which is counterintuitive.

Raw snacks are not the only way to sneak fresh vegetables into your diet. You can also steam or boil vegetables with your meals, for a quick, easy antioxidant punch. Instead of pouring that non-descript mush from the bag into a bowl and microwaving it, cut up some broccoli and asparagus and steam it in a pot. Top with hot butter and a pinch of salt and pepper, serve with your favorite protein, and you have a meal that is not only faster and more anti0xidant rich than before, but it is also probably cheaper too.

This sounds obvious, and it is, but it's vastly overlooked. The secret to consuming lots of fresh vegetables is having lots of fresh vegetables, and making them easy to access. Make sure you always have cut up veggies in your fridge, and some frozen veggies on hand, and add a little to every meal.

When you are feeling lazy, it is very easy to throw some frozen or cut up vegetables into your ready-made soup for a quick anti-oxidant boost. Alternatively, fresh veggies are great mixed into omelets or wraps.

Sometimes though, we all just want to sit back, put our feet up, watch

TV, and munch on something salty and crispy. Even I will admit, on these nights, carrot sticks will just not satisfy. If all you can think of is munching on a nice handful of chips, do not deny yourself; just remember the golden rule – EAT REAL FOOD! Instead of buying the giant discount bag of "crisps" with a 25-item ingredient list you can't pronounce, opt for the vegetable chips. There are many brands of chips these days that use carrots, jicama, sweet potato, and turnip instead of conglomerated chemicals. This way you can get the satisfying crunch while knowing you are boosting your antioxidants at the same time.

Fresh Fruits and Berries

Even if you hate the thought of vegetables, and you still make the same face you did when you were five when someone mentioned broccoli, you can still increase your antioxidant intake by other means, whilst you're adjusting to a more vegetable rich diet.

I have yet to meet someone who does not enjoy a sweet, juicy, ripe strawberry on a hot summer's day. That's not to suggest they aren't out there, but most people will have at least one favorite fruit. Luckily for us, fruits and berries are one of the best sources of antioxidants!

Again, the secret to consuming more fruits and vegetables is simply accessibility. When you set up your office or work space in the morning, make a little fruit bowl for you to snack on. It is easy to choose a ripe banana, a handful of sweet blackberries, or a slice of juicy mango over a chocolate bar, so long as you have that banana, those blackberries, or that mango, close by.

Alternatively, fruit salad is a cheap easy snack to prepare. Cut up your favorite fruits and berries, mix them together in a bowl, pour a thick dollop of low fat greek yogurt over top and there you have it – a Super Antioxidant Illness Fighting Snack.

If fresh fruits and veggies are not your thing, there are many prepared fruit bars and snacks at the grocery store. It is easy to choose a healthy fruit bar, or individually prepared fruit snack when they taste as good as these. Just remember to check the label for ingredients.

Finally, as long as you have access to a blender, a few fruits and vegetables, and some cream or dairy alternative, you can blend up your own healthy, antioxidant healing sherbet for dessert. Even your most picky, healthy-food abhorrent guest will love the rich taste of blended fruits and berries.

Remember, the more fruits and berries you eat, the more antioxidants you're likely to benefit from.

Whole Grains

Whole grains are an important, but often overlooked source of antioxidants.

Again, increasing your antioxidant consumption just comes down to EATING REAL FOOD. Most of us prepare some sort of carb, or grain with our meals, whether it is our oatmeal at breakfast, our sandwich bread at lunch, or out pasta for dinner, we eat a lot of grains, sometimes unknowingly.

Unfortunately, the most common store bought foods include only partial or artificial grains. To make sure you are consuming the healthier (and antioxidant rich) option, look out for whole grains in all your breads, pastas, and grains.

Some key words to look for while shopping are 'Whole Grains', 'Seven Grain', 'Ancient Grain', 'Quinoa', 'Flax', and 'Barley' to name a few.

You can also eat more whole grains by adding them to meals that you would not normally. Cooked and cooled quinoa is a great addition to a salad, and whole grain rice pudding is a unique and satisfying dessert.

Nuts and Legumes

Nuts and legumes are the often forgot about, antioxidant rich cousins to whole grains. Some nuts and legumes that are high in antioxidants are sunflower seeds, almonds, pumpkin seeds, hemp seeds, and walnuts.

Just like with fruits and vegetables, the easiest way to consume more nuts and legumes is to make them readily available. Make a trail mix with a variety of fresh nuts and legumes that you can snack on as you work and because of their rich but delicate flavor and satisfying crunch, nuts and legumes are easily added to many meals. Chopped nuts are as delicious on top of salad as they are on ice cream.

An easy way to sneak in nuts and legumes is to blend them in a food processor and replace the breadcrumbs or flour in your recipe with these powdered nuts and legumes. This way you get extra antioxidants without giving up your favorite recipe.

Finally, you will find a huge selection of sweet, chewy granola bars in the snack section of your local grocery store. As long as you are careful to read the label and avoid any confusing or scary sounding ingredients, granola bars can be a healthy, convenient way to sneak more antioxidants into your diet.

Dark Leafy Greens

Spinach. Swiss Chard. Beet Greens. Kale. These are hardly the ingredients we think of when imagining a delicious, satisfying meal. These dark leafy greens, however, are the Kings and Queens of antioxidant rich vegetables.

Salad, of course, is the go to vehicle to for those chanting "Eat your Greens, Eat your Greens!" And while I am right there with them chanting, I agree that raw swiss chard or kale can be hard stomach, especially for those vegetable-averse eaters.

Instead of trying to find ways to eat raw dark, leafy greens, I choose to sneak dark leafy greens into every meal.

In general, adding a handful of spinach or kale to a sauces, soups, or even omelets, will do little to affect the flavor of your dish. Instead, these greens will dramatically increase your antioxidant quotient for that meal. As an added bonus, a little green will make you look like a health-food guru compared to your fast-food toting neighbors.

Another easy way to sneak in dark antioxidant rich leafy greens is to simply replace any lettuce with something darker and richer. Where you might use iceberg or romaine lettuce in sandwiches or salads, use a darker, heartier leaf, like spinach. As well as adding vitamins and antioxidants, these dark leafy greens tend to be much stronger – this means they will not get soggy under salad dressings or sandwich spreads by the time you reach your lunch break.

Finally, do not underestimate the power of a little butter and garlic to ramp up any dish. While sautéing a variety of leafy greens may sound simple enough, when you had fresh butter, garlic, and herbs, you can easily create something deliciously decadent to serve alongside your main course.

As always, today's health craze has brought us many benefits, albeit a little stressful to try to wade through. You can find kale or beet-green chips in most health foods; these can be a healthy, satisfying way to sneak antioxidant rich leafy greens into your evening snack regime. And no need to feel guilty – every time you eat antioxidant rich foods you are adding extra arsenal to your body's illness fighting army.

Seek progression rather than perfection

This chapter (and book) has been written to help you take those all-important initial steps. My goals is to increase your awareness, and get your antioxidant intake higher than it was prior to reading this book. Don't be afraid to get creative with implementing healthy food into your diet and I encourage my friends and family to 'try something at least once' before judging it.

In the following chapter, we'll look at how you can increase your intake by drinking antioxidants.

THE TOP 3 WAYS TO DRINK YOUR ANTIOXIDANTS

Oftentimes we forget about beverages when we think of healthy eating. But the truth is, beverages can make up a big part of our daily consumption, and they can be just as detrimental or beneficial as the foods we eat. The good thing, though, is beverages tend to be a quicker and easier source of change than food.

Again going back to that Golden Rule, you should be thinking about what is in the beverages you are drinking. Just like you should EAT REAL FOOD, you should DRINK REAL THINGS.

Instead of reaching for miscellaneous concoctions for after work drinks, starting your day with chemical-laden expensive specialty coffees, or vending machine sodas, think about what is in these beverages. If you only drink beverages in which you know and understand the ingredients to be real; you will automatically increase your daily antioxidant consumption.

To start, the three beverages you should absolutely choose when you are feeling a little thirsty but also want to increase your antioxidants are; tea, smoothies and wine.

Tea

You do not have to tell me twice – caffeine is a gift from the gods! I can hardly open my eyes before I think about the wonderfully delicious jolt

I will feel after my first warm beverage settles in my belly. And while coffee might be popular the world over, tea is actually more affluent and an older cultural staple when looking at the whole of world history! An unlike coffee, tea is generally accepted in its most pure and beneficial form.

Although I would be hesitant to say natural, black coffee is bad for you, and in fact it is a source of antioxidants, natural black coffee is rarely what we see these days. Most often when people drink coffee in today's busy, capitalist society, they are drinking an expensive, chemically-laden concoction that is as far from true coffee as white chocolate is from the cacao bean. If not bought in a pretentious coffee house, coffee is usually served with one or all of the following fatty foods: cream, white sugar, or chocolate.

Tea, on the other hand, has survived the test of time. There is still a certain elegance and simplicity associated with a hot, relaxing cup of tea.

Black tea served at the start your day can provide an equal jolt as coffee does, but without the negative additives. As well, it tends to be higher in illness fighting antioxidants.

In the evening, a hot cup of green tea is just the thing to help you wind down after a hard day at the office. Fun fact: Green tea is so high in antioxidants; you can purchase green tea supplements at most health food stores, purely for the antioxidant dose. Natural green tea does contain caffeine, so be weary if you're taking it later into the evening.

In my opinion, though, the best part about black or green tea as an antioxidant supplement is its pure simplicity. It takes nothing more than a few tea leaves, a kettle of hot water, and your favorite tea cup to help you either start the day or wind down the evening while boosting your daily antioxidant consumption.

So take my advice, prepare yourself a cup of tea, and bask in the knowledge that you are helping your body fight off all kinds of illnesses and diseases.

Smoothies

Yum! Who does not love a fresh made smoothie – it blends the best of all worlds – creamy, rich, sweet, easy, and healthy. Best of all, you can include nearly all the antioxidant rich foods I mentioned in Chapter 1, in one easy to consume smoothie.

With enough natural yogurt, fruit juice and sweet berries, you can blend nearly anything into a smoothie and it will still taste like a milkshake: spinach, hemp seeds, bananas, cashews, apples, carrots – you name it, you can blend it.

The other great thing about smoothies is that they are so easy to prepare. You can pick up a decent blender at your local kitchen or second-hand store for under $20; after that all you need is fresh fruits and veggies, a few legumes, and a dairy or dairy alternative to give it a bit of creaminess, if you like that sort of thing.

It takes the same amount of time, or often less, to blend a smoothie as it does to scramble some eggs or butter and jam some toast. But, by adding so many antioxidant rich superfoods into one beverage, you are supercharging your body's ability to fight against illness and disease.

Wine

Last but not least, I could not finish the beverage section without mentioning my favorite of all beverages – wine.

While both white and red wine contain some antioxidants, I recommend red wine over white. Red wine tends to contain more antioxidants with less sugar, therefore making it superior to white wine in the race for antioxidant superfoods.

Red wine is so rich in antioxidants for the simple reason it is made from dark red grapes – belonging to one of the antioxidant rich food groups I mentioned in Chapter 1. As well, red wine is often blended with other antioxidant rich foods such as apples, nuts, and chocolate, thereby compounding its antioxidant potential.

Now, do not be mistaken, I am not encouraging gluttony in any sense. I am only saying that most of us enjoy relaxing with a tipsier beverage from time to time - when you are having friends over or celebrating your next promotion, choose red wine over prepared mixed drinks or carb-heavy beer to sneak antioxidants into even the most decadent of consumptions.

TREASURE HUNT – FIND ANTIOXIDANT FOOD SOURCES IN A FUN AND EASY WAY

As I said in the introduction, we are inundated on a daily basis with new instructions on what we should be eating, what we should be avoiding, what is good for us, and what is bad for us.

Yes, I understand the irony in my critique of the health industry when I myself have sat down and put finger to key to give you - the reader - advice on how to be your healthiest self. However, my goal is different in that I am only aiming to give you the fun, easy strategies to increase your antioxidants – the true warriors in your body's artillery against illness and disease.

So, rather than load you up with a bunch of fancy words, and a list of things to do and not do, I am going to give you an easy, familiar strategy to boost the antioxidants in your life.

Think of this as a Treasure Hunt of sorts – with the three strategies I give you, you will be able to make a fun antioxidant search out of every meal. Get the whole family involved! It is great to encourage your kids to start thinking about antioxidants at an early age, and with my simple strategy family members of any age can help out.

The secret Treasure Hunt is **R-R-R**! No, I am not talking about Rest, Relaxation, and Reduction, but those are important to good health too. And neither am I referring to Reduce, Reuse, Recycle, but I wholly encourage that as well (the topic of another book, perhaps). The Antioxidant **R-R-R** Treasure Hunt is: **Rainbow, Read, Rich**.

Rainbow

This category is a favorite for families with small children, since it helps them learn the colors of the rainbow, while also learning about antioxidant rich foods. One of the primary strategies of incorporating antioxidants into your diet is making sure you have a wide variety of different colored fruits, vegetables, berries, and other foods.

The Rainbow strategy is easy in that all you try to do is include as many colors of the rainbow into each meal as possible. If you have trouble remembering the colors of the rainbow, use the acronym **ROYGBIV** (rolls off the tongue doesn't it!):

R - Red

O - Orange

Y - Yellow

G - Green

B - Blue

I - Indigo

V - Violet

For example, a Rainbow Dinner might include:

R - Red Tomatoes

O - Orange Sweet Potatoes

Y - Yellow Spaghetti Squash

G - Green Spinach

B - Blue berries

I - Indigo Eggplant

P - Purple Cabbage

With this you could make Spaghetti Squash with cabbage, sweet potato, and eggplant in a spinach and tomato sauce, with blueberries and cream for dessert.

You do not necessarily need get every color of the rainbow in every meal, but by making this a goal you will naturally sneak more and more varieties of fruits and vegetables into every meal.

Let's try it again, but this time we will make a Rainbow Breakfast:

R - Red Strawberries

O - Oranges

Y - Yellow Bananas

G - Green Spinach

B - Blueberries

I – Indigo Currants

P - Purple Grapes

You could easily mix strawberries, oranges, bananas, spinach, blueberries, currants, and grapes in with a bit of yogurt to make a Super

Antioxidant Smoothie. Have this with a hot cup of black tea and you have the perfect start to the day.

Read

I have said it numerous times but I will say it again as the premise cannot be overstated, the best thing you can do for your body is EAT REAL FOOD. And how do you make sure you are eating real food? You READ THE LABEL!

A few rules to remember as you are reading the labels:

- If you can't pronounce it, it might not good for you.

- If you do not know what it is, you probably should not eat it.

- If there are more than 10-15 ingredients, you probably should not eat it.

- If the three out of the top five ingredients are sugar, it is probably not good for you.

When you are reading the labels, look for foods you recognize; foods you know to be good for you. Although chips are not generally thought of as a health food, if you read the label and see that these chips are made with sweet potato, kale, jicama, eggplant and salt, you should not feel guilty about eating them.

When you are out to eat at your favorite restaurant or fast food joint, make sure you read the whole menu. Often we choose items based on our familiarity with them, their proximity to where we are standing or sitting, or simply because that is what we chose last time. Instead, I encourage you to read the whole menu. Not only will you find new and interesting menu items, you will likely find options that are higher in antioxidants. And in my honest opinion, most foods that are higher in antioxidants are higher in flavor as well.

Read everything you eat. Read the label, read the ingredients, read the menu. If you can't read it, you probably should not eat it – simple as that!

Read Real Food → Eat Real Food

Rich

Last but not least, take the rich challenge every time you eat. No, I am not telling you to be rich in pocket – that would go against the very goal of this book to show you fun, easy, and affordable ways to sneak antioxidants into your diet.

Instead, I am talking about richness in food, richness in color, and richness in health. This is another good challenge for the whole family, because even the youngest of children can see that a Red Delicious apple has a richer color than a Granny Smith apple.

A general rule of thumb – the darker the fruit or vegetable, the more antioxidants are in the food. It is antioxidants and vitamins that give food that dark rich color.

This challenge is simple – look at the recipe you have in front of you, or the foods you are going to buy, or the items you are choosing between on the menu – once you are looking at these foods, see if you can think of a richer version of the foods you are eating, and swap them out.

For example, if you are making a salad with iceberg lettuce, yellow peppers, and chopped green apple, you can easily swap the iceberg lettuce for spinach, the yellow peppers for cooked sweet potato, and the chopped green apple for chopped red delicious apple. Just like that you have an equally, if not more, delicious salad, but with much healthier and more antioxidant rich foods.

For nearly every food you choose, there will be a richer alternative. The richer options are not only richer in antioxidants but also richer in taste and texture. I will give you a few examples of the richness challenge below. I will make a list of vegetables from the least rich to the richest, to show you how fun and easy this can be.

Iceberg Lettuce → Romaine Lettuce → Swiss chard → Spinach → Beet Tops → Kale

Celery →Cucumber → Zucchini → Green Pepper → Broccoli → Artichoke

White Grape → Red Grape → Strawberry → Raspberry → Blackberry → Fig → Currant

You see, just like that you can make your drinks and meals healthier and more antioxidant rich, as early as the grocery store. So get the whole family together and see who can make the richest, most antioxidant fueled meal!

Use the Antioxidant **R-R-R** Treasure Hunt to incorporate more antioxidants into every meal in a fun, family friendly, easy way. Get the whole family together and go on an Antioxidant Treasure Hunt for your next grocery trip!

TOP 10 CHEAP, HASSLE FREE AND ANTIOXIDANT RICH MEALS

I am not here to give you a list of do's and don'ts, and likewise, I do not plan of making this book a recipe book. I think I have given you the tools in the previous chapters that will enable you to go forth and make healthier, antioxidant conscious choices in your meal planning. That being said, I am not quite ready to let you off on your own just yet.

Below are my top ten cheap, hassle free, and most importantly, antioxidant rich, meal choices.

Fruit and Yogurt

Fruit and yogurt is one of the fastest, easiest, and most antioxidant rich meals you can start your day with. Here are the steps to making a delicious antioxidant rich fruit and yogurt breakfast:

- Look into your fridge and use the **R-R-R** method to choose the best fruits and berries to start your day.

- I suggest you choose a thick, low fat or sugar free Greek yogurt, but even generic berry flavored yogurt will be antioxidant rich.

- Choose a variety of nuts and seeds for your breakfast bowl. Look for nuts and seeds with good flavor and texture and throw in few dried berries: try pumpkin seeds, hemp seeds, chia, and dried date.

- Once you have chosen your ingredients, simply top the fruits and berries with your chosen yogurt, sprinkle with seeds and berries, and enjoy!

Omelets

Omelets are basically the stew of breakfast. It is so easy to make a delicious masterpiece out of whatever vegetable clippings are in your refrigerator at the time. Experiment with different grains such as quinoa to give your omelet a heartier texture and more staying power to fuel your day.

Try making a rainbow omelet:

R - Red Peppers
O - Orange Peppers
Y - Yellow Peppers
G - Green Spinach
B - Blue (Black) beans
I - Indigo cabbage
V - Violet (purple) Onion

Smoothies

Just like I said before, everyone loves a smoothie! Literally throw any fruits, vegetables, and leafy greens into your blender, add a bit of heavy yogurt or cream and maybe a dash of honey if you like things a little sweeter.

Salads

Although it may seem redundant, salads are of course one of the best sources of antioxidants in your daily meal. Use the 'Rich challenge', to make the most antioxidant rich salad you can. And do not limit yourself to vegetables. You can mix in all of the food groups I mentioned in Chapter 1 to make a delicious, filling, Antioxidant Super Salad.

I will list the ingredients of my favorite Antioxidant Super Salad below:

Spinach

Kale

Carrot

Red Peppers

Sweet Potatoes

Beets

Asparagus

Quinoa

Strawberries

Black Berries

Sunflower Seeds

Hemp Seeds

Dried cranberries

Pumpkin seeds

Goat Cheese

All drizzled in extra virgin olive oil and balsamic vinaigrette.

Wraps

Who are we kidding? A wrap is basically a salad in a tortilla, so take your favorite salad recipe, add some chicken, tuna, or your favorite protein, wrap it in a tortilla with some mustard and mayo and there you have another great antioxidant rich meal.

Sandwiches

Similar to wraps, sandwiches can be dressed up as far as your imagination will allow. I love to add roasted veggies and a variety of rich sprouts to my sandwiches. By adding a berry sauce, such as cranberry, and using a whole grain bread enriched with nuts and seeds, you will include all the antioxidant food groups in one easy to hold, playground classic lunch.

Pastas

By choosing whole grain pasta and making your own sauce with a variety of fresh, rainbow vegetables, you can make a quick, easy Antioxidant super food and spend less than you would if you ordered a pizza! And on a cold winter's day, nothing is quite as comforting as a hot steaming bowl of pasta.

Sauces

On the topic of pasta, make your own sauce. If you do not make your own, at least enrich yours with the extra vegetables you have in your fridge. It's easy to use the **R-R-R** method to spruce up any pasta sauce.

Pro tip: adding blended nuts such as almonds or cashews will thicken your homemade sauce, while giving it a deeper flavor and a great antioxidant boost!

Roasts

Roasts, the staple of an English Sunday lunch. Although I am sure you have gleaned from this book's emphasis on fast and simple, I am not one to slave over a hot stove all day making a giant feast. Besides, I would rather have more time to enjoy my next antioxidant boosting suggestion.

No, the roasts I am talking about are easy dishes of your choice of protein, surrounded by a variety of rainbow vegetable. Once you have everything in one big pot with a drizzle of olive oil and sprinkle of salt and pepper, throw everything into the oven to roast, and sit back and enjoy the aroma. Again, use the **R-R-R** Treasure Hunt method to choose a wide variety of rich, rainbow colored vegetables. Not only will your meal be antioxidant rich, it will be an impressive display as well.

Desserts

Desserts, most think, are the place where diets go to die. But that is the best part of my suggestion – I am not giving you a diet. I am simply giving you tools to make the healthiest possible decisions so that you can boost your body's antioxidant supply and fight of illness every day.

So, using everything you have learned in this book, an easy decision is made at dessert time. Instead of choosing the questionable frozen dessert, pulled out of a box half covered in unreadable ingredients, choose the single origin pure dark chocolate with a glass of rich red wine, and bask in the piece-of-mind that your dessert is actually benefitting your health, unlike the others in the room.

FOOD & DRINK-FREE ANTIOXIDANT BOOSTERS

While it goes without saying that the focus of this book is to help you increase antioxidants into your everyday diet in an effortless way, it would not be complete without affording you some suggestions on how to boost your antioxidants without food or drink… even in your sleep.

Go back to the introduction of this book, where I explained to you what an antioxidant is. Remember, an antioxidant stops free radicals in your body, by stopping the oxidation (or unchanging) of your cells.

By looking at the natural causes of oxidation, we can learn the lifestyle choices we should make to boost our body's natural antioxidant production. Some causes of oxidation in the body are pollution, stress, over-exertion, and cigarette smoke. The main lifestyle choices we can make to increase antioxidants in our bodies stem from these causes of oxidation:

Rest

The first and foremost lifestyle change we can make to encourage our body's antioxidant production is to rest. Too often we are rushing from work to home, to the grocery store, to a friend's house, and then back home. When do we ever rest? Our bodies need time to wind down from the constant rush of everyday life.

Set aside at least half an hour everyday where you will allow yourself to rest. This is a time where your body and mind are calm, and you can recharge. Some people choose meditation; others sleep; you might embroider. Whatever you choose, make sure you mind and body are relaxed and you are wholly present in the moment.

Light Exercise

Over-exertion is a cause of oxidative stress in the body, but our bodies absolutely need some exercise to stay healthy. Keep your activity light to moderate, so that your heart rate is rising a little bit, but you are not out of breath.

Some easy, fun activities that incorporate light exercise into your routine are walking, gardening, dancing, yoga or canoeing. There are literally 1,000's to choose from. The key to light exercise is to move your body so you're breathing rate and heart rate increase, whilst not considering it 'exercise'. Find an activity that you enjoy.

Reduce Stress

Numerous studies have shown that stress has an irreversible negative effect on all parts of your body. To ensure your body can adequately produce antioxidants, try to reduce your stress levels. This might mean you lessen your workload at the office, take part in activities that you can relax and enjoy or ask for help from your partner during high stress times at home.

If your heart rate is rising or you are having trouble sleeping, you might be stressed. Take a look at your life and see if there are any ways you can reduce your stress levels.

Remember, there is no shame in asking for help. Ask a friend, family member, or health practitioner about ways you can limit your stress.

Sleep More

As we are told so often, sleep is vital to healthy living! Is your TV show really worth staying up for? Are you trying to sleep on old lumpy pillows? Make sleep a priority in your life, if you want your body to produce the most antioxidants possible.

The best part about these food and drink free lifestyle antioxidant boosters is that you can incorporate all of them into one. Going for a long but light stroll after work will help you to de-stress while you get light exercise. When you get home you will be calm, rested, and ready for a good night's sleep.

SUPER ANTIOXIDANT BREAKFAST, LUNCH AND DINNER OPTIONS

Now you have all the tools you need to make healthy choices in meal, drink and lifestyle, leading you to an antioxidant rich life.

Remember, eating antioxidants can be fun, easy, and affordable. Simply use the **R-R-R** Treasure Hunt when choosing drinks and meals, and get lots of rest.

If you eat real food you, drink real things, and live for the real you, you are guaranteed to be rich in antioxidants.

And if you are rich in antioxidants you will be rich in fighting power against illnesses such as Parkinson's disease, Alzheimer's disease, cancer, neurodegenerative disorders, auto immune disorders, and more.

So here, I leave you with 5 Super Antioxidant additions for breakfast, lunch and dinner:

Breakfast

- Omelet with leafy greens
- Berries with yogurt and seeds
- Fruit salad with yogurt

- Berry and greens smoothie

- Whole grain hot cereal with berries and seeds

Lunch

- Roasted vegetable sandwich with berry sauce

- Mixed raw vegetable wrap

- Hearty salad with seeds, grains and berries

- Vegetable soup with whole grain bread

- Mixed Vegetables on top of whole grains

Dinner

- Roasted vegetables and protein

- Hearty Vegetable soup with whole grain bread

- Steamed Vegetable Pasta

- Marinated Vegetable Stew

- Sautéed leafy greens over whole grains and roasted vegetables

CONCLUSION

If you frequently go to health stores or a friend tells you all about their detox diet, you may hear antioxidants come up a lot of the time and for very good reason! They are packed with invaluable benefits that will help to protect you from environmental damage to just helping your body replenish its cells. Either way, not getting enough of the antioxidants listed in the book will take a toll on your body and health, maybe not right away but progressively, you'll start to see the effects.

When it comes to food, nourishment is key. Unfortunately most people go for convenience and a low price tag. It's prioritizing your health over being lazy and not wanting to put the effort into taking care of yourself. Everyone has time.

Not only that but antioxidants play a vital role in aging; of the skin and of the cells. When your cells die instead of replenish, these show up on the skin as aging. This is often because healthy cells are not supposed to die and if your body can't recognize harmful cells, it's mostly due to your diet.

As the genius Warren Buffett once said; 'Knowing that I had only one car that had to last a lifetime, what would I do with it? I would read the manual about 5 times, I would always keep it garaged, if there was the least little dent or scratch, I'd have it fixed right away because I wouldn't want it rusting. I would baby that car because it would have to last a lifetime'.

That's exactly how you should treat yourself. You only get one body and one mind and it has to last a lifetime. It's very easy to let them ride for many years but after that, 40 years later it will be a wreak. It's what you do right now that will determine the condition of your mind and body, 10, 20 or 30 years down the line.

By implementing even 20% of what this book offers, you'll be making a concerted effort to increasing antioxidants into your body, improving your body's natural defense system and enhancing your life.

I hope that I've demonstrated that the process doesn't have to be difficult, boring or expensive. Take that step to improving the only body you will ever have TODAY. It doesn't have to be life changing amounts straight away, but just commit to continually increasing your antioxidant levels day by day and week by week. Your body and mind will repay you ten-fold.

ABOUT THE AUTHOR

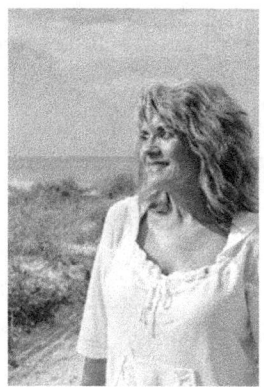

Ruth Logan has been fascinated with Personal Development, Health, and Wellbeing for just over 30 years now. She's particularly passionate about Eastern Philosophy, and the Science behind Wellbeing. Her aim is to share the great benefits of Eastern Philosophy to the unaware in modern society.

Ruth is an avid reader and can't resist learning new information on how we can all better ourselves. Over the last couple of years she's started freelance writing and more recently taken the step to releasing her on work.

In her books, Ruth provides action plans and advice on how to incorporate learning points into 'real life' in a concise yet informative manner.

When not reading or writing, Ruth enjoys walking her dog, cooking and travel.

MORE BOOKS BY

RUTH LOGAN

If you enjoyed reading "**Antioxidants**", you may like these other books from Ruth Logan.

Beauty Bath – How to Create a Professional Quality Home Spa for Relaxation and Pure Indulgence

Gratitude – 7 Simple Steps To Becoming More Grateful In 7 Days

Healing – 7 Ways To Heal Your Body in 7 Days

Learning – 7 Steps To Increasing Your Learning Your Learning Potential In 7 Days

Limiting Beliefs – 7 Ways To Stop Limiting Beliefs In 7 Days

Aromatherapy – A Beginner's Guide To Using Aromatherapy At Home